Ultimate Carb Cycling Guide!

Carb Cycling

Quickly Lose Fat, Preserve Muscle Mass, And Build Self Confidence With Sustainable Fat Loss Carb Cycling Diet Tips And Strategies That Work Fast!

I0417003

Chris Smith

Legal Notice

Disclaimer Notice

Table Of Contents

Introduction

I want to thank you and congratulate you for purchasing the book, *Carb Cycling: Ultimate Carb Cycling Guide! - Quickly Lose Fat, Preserve Muscle Mass, And Build Self Confidence With Sustainable Fat Loss Carb Cycling Diet Tips And Strategies That Work Fast!*

This book contains proven steps and strategies on how to plan your own carb cycling diet with explanations of the concept, the science behind it, and several food recommendations.

Have you heard of cyclic ketogenic diet? No? Well, that isn't a bad thing. You probably already know about it, more popularly known as carb cycling.

To keep one's body fit, there are a lot of things to consider. One of those is attaining an ideal weight. If you already have an ideal weight, then it's just a matter of maintaining it. If you're overweight, then you have to reduce weight. If you're underweight, then you should gain weight. But you shouldn't just stop with the numbers you see on the weighing scale. Your body's composition is also important. When losing or gaining weight, you must be sure that you are losing fat and gaining muscle.

Two things play the greatest part here: diet and physical activity. Weight is about the calories: how much you get from the food you eat and how much you spend on the physical things you do. There should be a correct balance between them. Diet and exercise go hand in hand in this matter. Although these two things can be discussed together, our main focus here is dieting.

Chapter 1: Understand The Concept Of Carb Cycling

There have been a lot of diets formulated since long ago. You probably heard of many whether you've been searching or not. To a certain extent, all of them can work since diet is basically calorie deficit. Consume less than what you spend and you lose weight. The thing is that a healthy weight is not just about the quantity but also the quality. It is not just how much you eat that matters, but also the kind of food you eat. Diet can get a little complicated especially if you have further goals such as building and toning your muscles or gaining an ideal body for a specific sport.

Carb cycling is one of the many diets popular among body-builders and athletes. That's because it can build and maintain muscle mass. Also, it adds efficiency in fat burning.

Carb cycling may have its roots from bodybuilding but now it gained significance even in the general health community. That explains a good part of why it's getting a great deal of attention nowadays. Since you're reading this book, it's quite likely that it got your attention, too. You probably want an in-depth learning of carb cycling. So, let's finish up this introduction and get to the good part: learning about carb cycling and how to apply it.

In order to effectively apply carb cycling into your own lifestyle, you must understand deeply its concept. As mentioned earlier, the science behind the diet can get really complicated. But don't worry. You don't really need to go into all the technical terms and whatnot in order to understand carb cycling, or any diet for that matter. This book will still discuss the science behind carb cycling but it can be simplified enough for the average person.

What is carb cycling?

Controlling carbohydrate intake has been of great importance when talking about nutrition. Studies abound regarding the relation of improper carbohydrate intake to serious health concerns such as chronic diseases and obesity. But still, carbohydrates are also important for our body. So, it is not always just about reducing the carbohydrates you consume, but actually taking in the right amount of carbohydrates.

The above is the reason why carb cycling and similar diets were formed. The carb cycling diet uses an approach of alternating the level of carbohydrate consumption. Such a diet involves periods of zero, low and high carbohydrate intake. As it turns out, it isn't just about taking in the right kind and amount of carbohydrates but also taking them at the right time. The kind of carbohydrates, how much, and when you will take them influence how your body responds to them.

In a carb cycling diet, you schedule your week into no-carb, low-carb, and high-carb days. Note that a high-carb day doesn't mean you'll pig out on carbs – you still control the amount but just higher compared to the other days. You'll see more on that later.

A carb cycling diet doesn't only take carbs into consideration. There's also protein and fat – taking the right amount of these is equally important. Throughout the schedule, you need a high level of protein intake. For fat, it is inversely proportional to your carb intake. Thus, during zero or low-carb days, your fat intake should be high. During high-carb days, you consume low fat.

Carb cycling diets will be varied in terms of specific protocols. However, they all share the same basis. The structure is simple: a few days of low-carbs, one day of high-carbs, followed by a day of zero-carbs or low-carbs, and the cycle goes back to the beginning.

As an example, you may schedule four consecutive days of low-carb, high-carb the next day, zero-carb after that, and back to the beginning. Or, schedule three consecutive days of low-carb, one high-carb day, and then back to low-carb.

To gain insight on what is involved in a carb cycling diet, here are some numerical figures:

- On a high-carb day, your set amount of carbohydrate intake is generally between 2 to 2.5 grams for every pound of body weight. Protein intake is set at 1 gram for every pound while fat intake is set to 0 to 0.15 grams for every pound.

- On a moderate-carb day, carbohydrate intake is 1.5 grams for every pound. Protein is at 1 to 1.2 grams for every pound, and fat is at 0.2 grams for every pound.

- On a low-carb day, the intake is at 1.5 grams of carbohydrates for each pound of weight. Protein intake is generally increased to around 1.5 grams per body pound, and fat goes up to 0.35 grams for every pound.

- A zero-carb or no-carb day doesn't really mean zero carbohydrates at all. The term is just for distinguishing from the low-carb since the no-carb day has a really low limit. It no longer takes into consideration body weight – you must not go over 30 grams of carbohydrates for the whole day. Here, you consume 1.5 grams of protein for every pound and fat rises up to 0.5 to 0.8 grams for every pound. Note that this zero/no-carb day is skipped by some people. It is up to your goals or what fits your level of physical activity.

As you can see, the diet involves a detailed measurement of the carbohydrates, protein, and fat that you consume. It takes a lot of discipline especially if you have specific goals. You must really get into the diet if you want to accomplish it. However, once you start, you'll find that it is not as difficult to incorporate to your daily lifestyle compared to other types of diet. Furthermore, this book is a good starting point.

Chapter 2: The Science Behind Carb Cycling

How does carb cycling work?

It's time to get into the science behind carb cycling. In this part, we will make it clear how carb cycling works and clear some misconceptions. While anecdotes might be true or substantial, they aren't as reliable as Science. Furthermore, there is information out there that exaggerates or discredits carb cycling. Every false piece of information does not help in properly understanding how the diet really works.

The alternating level of carb consumption creates a different effect for your body. During the high-carb day in the cycle, the glycogen levels in your muscles are replenished and insulin production in your body is triggered. Insulin inhibits the breakdown of muscle cells. This is called anti-catabolic effects. Note that one closely because some people that discuss carb cycling may mislead you. There are claims that it has real anabolic effects – meaning it stimulates protein synthesis. Those are not true. However, while it doesn't cause protein synthesis, inhibiting muscle breakdown is enough to aid in losing weight and building muscle.

Moving on, we have the moderate-carb days. When consuming the moderate amount of carbs, you get enough for the maintenance of glycogen stores. But you also don't enter a caloric deficit to make you lose weight.

The low-carb and no-carb days are the ones that put you into a caloric deficit. Advocates who over-glorify carb cycling will tell you that these parts of the cycle does some "magic." Again, that is not true. Carb cycling works because of science. There's nothing magical about it. But while it is not magical, it is indeed effective. During these parts of the cycle, the insulin level in your body becomes low. The response of your body is to burn fat faster.

Now, this book is about diet, but it is important to touch a little about exercise. You already know that diet alone does not make a person physically fit. When it comes to carb cycling, you will also need to coordinate your exercise with the schedule.

The basic concept is really simple. On high-carb days, you perform your toughest workout. On moderate-carb days, you do your normal training. On low-carb or no-carb days, you rest or only do cardio. The specific calculations are more complicated. That's a topic for another book.

Caloric Deficit

Caloric deficit means you consume less energy than what your body spends. This is the root of any diet that aims for weight loss. Whether you put yourself in a caloric deficit on a daily, weekly, or monthly basis, it will make you lose weight. It doesn't matter whether you break down your macronutrient intake or not.

Carb cycling also uses caloric deficit. But another thing you'll hear from those glorifying carb cycling is that there's no need to count calories. They'll claim that you only have to follow the high-moderate-low cycling. This might work decent enough for maintenance or make you lose weight to a certain extent. But when it comes to extreme weight reduction, such a method will never be enough.

A crucial part of a carb cycling is taking the right amount of carbs, protein, and fat for your body. That means you have to accurately measure how much of these nutrients you are consuming when undergoing such a diet. So, don't believe anyone who says such is not necessary for carb cycling to work for significant weight loss. There's no scientific proof for that claim.

The thing to get from this chapter is that, yes, carb cycling works but it is not in any way a magic button that will get you your dream body in a snap. Carb cycling requires discipline and a high level of accuracy. Plus, you should carefully pair it with your training routine.

Chapter 3: Starting Carb Cycling (Scaling From A Previous Low-Carb Diet)

Now that you know what carb cycling is and the science behind it, let's address a question that you might have.

"How do I start carb-cycling? Also, can I start immediately?"

You can absolutely start carb cycling right away. But it might be quite difficult. If you are confident you can handle it, then, by all means do it. Otherwise, the recommended thing for you is to slowly scale your diet.

If you are already on a low carb diet, it would be easier for you. That's because you have already conditioned yourself to control your carb intake.

You begin by determining your body fat levels and then determining your goals. You have to be realistic of course. Maybe you want to achieve your ideal weight fast but the sudden change in diet might prove difficult for you. So, you have to weigh your options. If you need to cut down a lot of weight, there would be minimal carbs in your diet. But you need not hurry yourself if you don't want to. It might actually work better for you if you do it in a way that wouldn't be too inconvenient for you. It's easier to slowly build up the discipline instead of just diving in and giving up when it proves to be too much.

One thing you shouldn't forget is to continue your workout. You shouldn't reduce the intensity. Doing so will make the diet work better.

Plan your schedule. You aren't cycling yet so the amount of your carb intake every day is erratic. Based on the numerical figures discussed earlier, determine the ideal carb intake for you in the different stages in the cycle. Once you have crunched the numbers, gauge whether you can pull it off. In most cases, the concern is on the low-carb and no-carb days. Can you handle such a low intake? Yes? Then, that's good. No? Well, don't fret. You can start slow. Don't set the amount of carbs like the results in the computation yet. As you go through the cycles, slowly diminish the amounts until you get to the ideal intake.

In case you are already on a low-carb diet, then your intake would be the same every day. Like what's discussed above, take the ideal intake for you and set your cycle. If you've been doing the diet for a while, you will be quite good at controlling your cravings and measuring your intake. The probable problem is that you are so used to taking in low carbs that you are hesitant to do the high carb days. If so, just scale it slowly. Increase the intake for the high carb days and decrease it for the low carb days in small increments. This would be easier for you and won't be that hard to track.

Remember to stick to your planned schedule. Don't break the cycle. You might get really good at controlling carbs, and when you feel the desire to lose weight faster, you might get tempted to extend your low carb and no carb days. There is danger in doing so. You risk hurting yourself while training because of the low energy. In the long run, you may also cause damage to your body.

Chapter 4: Foods To Eat, Foods To Avoid

Now that you have been acquainted with scaling your current diet into a carb cycling diet, it's time to learn what food to eat and what to avoid. This is because there are different kinds of carbohydrates, proteins, and fats that you can get from the food you eat. A carb-cycling diet requires you to measure the exact amounts of these nutrients that you take. However, it's not just about the quantity. You also need to mind the quality.

Carbohydrates

Let's start with carbs. Carbohydrates are the body's primary source of energy. Whatever diet, they are an integral part in keeping your body healthy. That's why they should always be a part of your diet. Only, carbs aren't created equal.

There are simple and complex carbs. This is determined by their chemical composition and how the body processes them. In general, complex carbohydrates are better than simple ones. This is because complex carbs take longer for your body to break down so they provide even energy. But this isn't ideal in the context of carb-cycling. Simple carbs are easier to digest so it would be used fast as you work out. But in many cases, they just don't provide real value for your body. So, choosing the right carbohydrates for carb-cycling isn't just a matter of choosing between simple and complex carbs. There are other factors that come in as to what makes certain carbs ideal while others should be avoided.

Fruits and vegetables contain simple carbohydrates – simple sugars. What makes them different is that they are high in fiber. Fiber alters the way how the human body breaks down the carbs they contain. That makes them good sources of carbohydrates.

There are more scientific details about the factors that make certain carbohydrates good or bad. But we won't go through them all at length. For this book's purposes, a list of the foods to eat and foods to avoid would be enough. There will be brief explanations following some of the items.

Good Carbs

Here are good carb sources for a carb cycling diet.

- Milk – It has lactose, a good simple carb. Just be sure that you go for low-fat or zero-fat milk so you don't throw of the fat consumption part of your diet.

- White or Sweet Potato – Potatoes can satiate you faster, meaning you feel full faster, especially when boiled. The carbs are simple and they contain fiber.

- Fruits – The reasons have been touched already. Carbs are especially good for berries.

- Quinoa – This is really nice for the high carb days. You'll need starchy carbs like what quinoa has during these days in the cycle.

- Oatmeal

- Whole Grain Bread

- Tortillas

- Whole Wheat Pasta

- Brown Rice

Bad Carbs

Many foods contain junk carbs. Here are some things that you have to avoid when under a carb cycling diet.

- Pastries (such as doughnuts)

- Instant oatmeal (as they tend to contain a lot of sugar)

- Pizza

- Cookies, cakes, and the like

- Muffins and Croissants

Fats

Selecting fats you consume is also crucial to make a carb cycling diet work. Trans fats and saturated fats are bad. They raise cholesterol in your body which causes arteries to harden making you more prone to cardiovascular diseases. Polyunsaturated and monounsaturated fats, on the other hand, are good. They aid in lowering your cholesterol levels, in turn lowering the chances of contracting heart disease. Moreover, they improve the efficiency of insulin.

Good Fat

Here are some foods with good fat.

- Vegetable oil, olive oil, and other plant-based oils – If you'll need oil for cooking, then it's best to use these.

- Avocado

- Sunflower Seeds

- Herring, Mackerel, Trout, Sardines, Tuna, and Salmon, along with other fatty cold-water fish

- Walnuts and Flaxseed

Bad Fat

Here are foods that contain bad fats.

- Animal-based oils

- High-fat dairy products

- Red Meat

- Poultry Skin

- Some vegetable oils (like palm oil and coconut oil)

- French Fries and Potato Chips

- Microwaved Popcorn

- Most Frozen Foods

- Store-bought Baked Goods

- Egg Yolk

Proteins

"Carb" might be in the name of the diet, but proteins can be considered its real "star." Whatever day in the cycle, you got to take in a lot of protein. Proteins build up the muscles, aid in shedding unwanted weight, and keep your tummy full (ergo, keep you from overeating). Moreover, they also serve as building blocks to make your heart, bones, skin, and hair healthy – no matter if you're a bodybuilder or not. Of course, like the two previously discussed nutrients, you must take the right kind of protein. Here are some recommended sources that will fill your protein needs for a carb cycling diet.

- White meat (Poultry) – Poultry meat contains a good deal of protein and little fat. Just take off the skin.

- Milk and other dairy products – Just be careful to choose low-fat variants. They aren't only good sources of protein but also provide calcium.

- Seafood – They are recommended because of their low fat content. Some fish already mentioned above have higher fat but they are good fat.

- Soy – High in protein and aids in reducing cholesterol.

- Eggs – One egg a day is good. It has a good amount of protein. Going over that is not a good idea because of the fat.

- Pork Tenderloin – This is another type of white meat and contains lean protein.

- Lean Beef – The fat content is considerably low (comparable to a chicken breast with no skin). It also contains other important nutrients like vitamin B12, iron, and zinc.

- Beans –They contain a good deal of protein plus they have lots of fiber.

- Protein Powder –They are specially formulated so you can get the right amount of protein efficiently and conveniently.

Chapter 5: Planning Your Own Carb Cycling Diet

We went through a lot of recommendations. Now, we move to some guide. You can plan your very own carb cycling diet by following these steps.

1. Set your goals. How much weight do you want to lose? How low do you want your body fat percentage to drop? You must establish the aforementioned things exactly.

2. Choose your cycle. There are a few samples in the earlier chapter on what is carb cycling. Here's another: alternating between high carb and low carb days over six days and set the seventh day for "reward meals."

3. Calculate the amounts for the nutrient intake for each of the days in the cycle. How much protein, fats, and carbs must you take during low carb days? High carb days? You have seen previously that these amounts would depend on your current weight in pounds. The recommended amounts are given with a range except for the no carb day. Choose your number according to your goals.

4. Choose your food. They will serve as your fuel. The sizes of your servings depend on your calculated amounts and established schedule. The recommended foods are in the precious chapter. Stock your refrigerator with them.

5. Create your meal plan. It is best to plan different meals to give your cycles variety. It won't do you good if you make it more difficult by taking in the same food. So, just set the amounts and substitute meals in the plan.

Here are samples of plans for men and women taking into account high-carb and low-carb days.

For males

High-carb day:

- Protein – 1-1.25 grams for each pound of body weight

- Carbs – 2-3 grams for each pound of body weight

- Fat – the smallest amount possible

Low-carb day:

- Protein – 1.25-1.5 grams for each pound of body weight

- Carbs – 0.5-1.5 grams for each pound of body weight

- Fat – 0.15-0.35 grams for each pound of body weight

For females

High-carb day:

- Protein – 0.75 grams for each pound of body weight

- Carbs – around 1 gram for each pound of body weight

- Fat – the smallest amount possible

Low-carb day:

- Protein – around 1 gram for each pound of body weight

- Carbs – 0.2-0.5 grams for each pound of body weight

- Fat – 0.1-0.2 grams for each pound of body weight

Chapter 6: Low Carb Substitutes

One of the most difficult things about carb cycling and other diets that involve low carb intake is giving up food that have been "staple" on your previous diets. But you'll definitely need to do so because they are the heaviest carb contributor in your diet. The challenge is to find those low-carb foods that you can substitute for the high-carb ones. Here are some suggestions:

For Breads

Some people think that they can't live without bread. We can put in a Bible verse here but that's in a different context. Anyway, if you really love bread, there are low-carb alternatives, like:

- Low-carb bread – be sure to read the labels thoroughly

- Tortillas – low-carb ones

- Crisp breads – high in fiber

- Bread with low glycemic load – meaning your body converts the carbs in them more slowly than ordinary bread

For Pasta

Lots of tasty pasta meals are floating around restaurants and homes. Well, pasta is a high source of carbs. If you love them, here are some alternatives:

- Low-carb pasta

- Shirataki noodles

- Spaghetti squash

Also note that when you cook 100% whole grain pasta in a way that it is still slightly firm (called "al dente" by Italians), the pasta will have a low glycemic load. Such in small servings would be good to incorporate in your moderate or high carb days.

For Cereals

Many people might equate cold cereals with breakfast. They are easy to prepare so busy people and children love them. It's quite likely that you are fond of cereals. The problem with cereals is that they are generally too processed. As a result, their glycemic factors are high. Here are some alternatives:

- Low-carb cold cereals – they are available but might be hard to find.

- High-fiber cereals – still, check the labels and stay away from flavored ones

- Flax seed meal

- Ricotta cheese

For Rice

Rice might not be that big of a concern in the USA but in certain Asian countries, rice is staple food. If you eat rice regularly, it's one of the foods you have to give up during low-carb days. Then, for high carb days, opt for brown rice instead of the usual white rice. Brown rice has a lower glycemic load.

For Potato

Among unprocessed foods, one is known to have a high glycemic load: potatoes. If you love putting potatoes into your cooking or simply love mashed potatoes, you need alternatives. Well, there's no absolutely perfect alternative for potatoes, but with a little getting used to, some substitutes will work:

- Mashed cauliflower

- Celery root aka celeriac

- Other root crops with low carb content

- "instant mashers" – commercial products that are meant to be used like mashed potatoes

Chapter 7: 10 Delicious Protein Shake/Smoothie Recipes

One of the best ways to get your protein requirements in your carb cycling diet is via protein shakes or protein smoothies. They are portable and easy to prepare. Some people will dismiss them because they don't taste good. That is just wrong. With the right recipes, protein shakes can be delicious. Here are some recipes for healthy and delicious protein shakes/smoothies.

The Sunrise Smoothie

The first one is an ideal smoothie for breakfast – The Sunrise Smoothie.

Ingredients:

- 1 banana (frozen)

- 1 cup of mixed berries (organic, frozen)

- 1 orange (peeled, segmented)

- 4-6 oz Vanilla Greek Yogurt

Preparation:

1. Pour in all ingredients in your blender.

2. Blend until mixture becomes smooth or you get your desired texture.

The main protein source here is the Greek Yogurt. Aside from giving you 15 grams of protein, this smoothie also provides vitamin C (from the orange) and potassium (from the banana). It's a really good way to start your day.

Dark Chocolate Peppermint Protein Shake

The next one is more for snacking. It's called Dark Chocolate Peppermint Protein Shake.

Ingredients:

- 2-3 ice cubes

- 1 banana (frozen)

- 1 cup milk (non-dairy)

- 1 scoop whey protein powder of choice

- ¼ teaspoon peppermint extract (pure)

- 2 tablespoons high quality cocoa powder

- Pinch of sea salt

- Optional: 1 tablespoon chocolate chips (dark or vegan)

- Toppings: vegan whipped topping, Greek yogurt, home-made whipped cream

Preparation:

1. Pour in all ingredients in your blender.

2. Blend until mixture becomes smooth or you get your desired texture.

3. Pour in a tall glass and top with your choice of toppings.

For chocolate lovers who want to keep it healthy, this recipe would be really great. Main source of protein is the protein powder. Dark chocolate has a good amount of antioxidants.

Honey Banana Smoothie

The next one is pretty simple – the Honey Banana Smoothie.

Ingredients:

- 1 banana (frozen)

- 1 cup Greek Yogurt (plain, non-fat)

- 1 teaspoon honey

- 1 cup orange juice

- Nutmeg

Preparation:

1. Pour in all ingredients in your blender except the nutmeg.

2. Blend until mixture becomes smooth or you get your desired texture.

3. Pour in a tall glass and top with a pinch of finely grated nutmeg.

Again, we have the Greek Yogurt as the main protein source. The honey provides a healthy sweetener.

Chocolate Espresso Protein Smoothie

Next, we have the Chocolate Espresso Protein Smoothie.

Ingredients:

- 1 scoop chocolate protein powder

- ½ cup chilled brewed coffee or 1 teaspoon instant coffee grounds

- 1 teaspoon cocoa powder (high quality, non-sweetened)

- 1 cup coconut milk

- 1 banana (frozen, chunked)

- Optional: ½ cup ice

Preparation:

1. Mix the ingredients in a blender.

2. Blend until mixture becomes smooth or you get the desired texture.

The protein powder is the main protein source. Banana again provides potassium.

Green Vanilla Almond Shake

Want a post-workout shake? Try the Green Vanilla Almond Shake.

Ingredients:

- 1 cup ice

- 1 scoop protein powder

- 1 banana (frozen)

- 2 tablespoons almond butter

- 2 teaspoons vanilla extract (organic)

- 2 cups baby spinach

Preparation:

1. Mix the ingredients in a blender.

2. Blend until mixture becomes smooth or you get the desired texture.

You get the protein mainly from the powder and the almond butter. Spinach provides other substantial nutrients. Don't worry if you don't like its taste, the banana, vanilla, coconut milk, and protein powder masks it.

Strawberry Almond Protein Smoothie

You might have noticed that each recipe we discussed so far uses banana. Here's the first smoothie on our list without one – Strawberry Almond Protein Smoothie.

Ingredients:

- 1 cup strawberries (organic, frozen)

- ½ cup water (distilled)

- ½ cup almonds (soaked – ideally overnight)

Preparation:

1. Mix the ingredients in a blender.

2. Blend until mixture becomes smooth or you get the desired texture.

Almonds provide protein as well as other nutrients like manganese, iron, calcium, and zinc. Strawberries provide a nice spin to the taste as well as some vitamins.

Orange Mango Smoothie

Next is the Orange Mango Smoothie.

Ingredients:

- 1 scoop protein powder (vanilla, vegan)

- 1 cup mango chunks (frozen)

- 1 orange (peeled, segmented)

- 1 ½ cups almond milk (unsweetened)

- 2 tablespoons cashews

- 1 teaspoon cinnamon

- ½ teaspoon tumeric

Preparation:

1. Mix the ingredients in a blender.

2. Blend until mixture becomes smooth or you get the desired texture.

This smoothie is also nice for breakfast. The protein powder and cashews provide the protein. You get vitamin C from the orange. What makes this smoothie unique though is the tumeric. It might sound odd to add a spice into a shake, but the resulting taste is nice. Plus, tumeric contains a good amount of antioxidants.

Peanut Butter and Jelly Smoothie

The next one would satisfy the child in you. It's called Peanut Butter and Jelly Smoothie.

Ingredients:

- 1 cup berries (frozen)

- 1 tablespoon peanut butter (all-natural)

- 1 scoop whey protein powder

- 2 tablespoons oats (rolled)

- 1 cup soy milk

Preparation:

1. Mix the ingredients in a blender.

2. Blend until mixture becomes smooth or you get the desired texture.

You get a good deal of protein from the whey powder and peanut butter. It's like having your tasty bread filling in a healthy way as you skip the bread. The mixture of rolled oats, berries, and peanut butter provides a satisfying taste for the kid in you.

Green Warrior Protein Smoothie

Another green smoothie is coming up. Here's the Green Warrior Protein Smoothie.

Ingredients:

- 4 tablespoons hemp hearts

- 1 cup lacinato or dinosaur kale (destemmed)

- ½ cup grapefruit juice (fresh)

- 1 sweet apple (chopped, cored)

- 1 cucumber (chopped)

- ¼ cup mango chunks (frozen)

- ½ cup celery (chopped)

- 1/8 cup mint leaves (fresh)

- 3 cups ice cubes

- Optional: ½ tablespoon virgin coconut oil

- Optional: ½ tablespoon algae oil

Preparation:

1. Mix the ingredients in a blender except the algae oil (if using).

2. Blend until mixture becomes smooth or you get the desired texture.

3. Take the algae oil separately.

The hemp hearts provide a good deal of protein and also contains a nice amount of fiber. The fruits provide vitamins and makes the shake creamy and sweet.

Almond and Cookie Butter Oatmeal Protein Shake

Last but not the least is the Almond and Cookie Butter Oatmeal Protein Shake. It's nice for either breakfast or snacks.

Ingredients:

- 1 cup almond milk

- 2 cups ice cubes

- 1 scoop protein powder

- ¼ cup rolled oats

- 2 tablespoons cookie butter

- 3 tablespoons almond butter

- Pinch of cinnamon

Preparation:

1. Mix the ingredients in a blender.

2. Blend until mixture becomes smooth or you get the desired texture.

Protein mainly comes from the protein powder and almond butter. The cookie butter provides the nice taste.

Conclusion

The book provided you with the information you need in order to plan your own carb cycling diet. I hope you have enjoyed it and learned some new ideas or tips. Just one new tip or piece of advice can change everything!

Thank you again for purchasing the book Carb Cycling: Ultimate Carb Cycling Guide! - Quickly Lose Fat, Preserve Muscle Mass, And Build Self Confidence With Sustainable Fat Loss Carb Cycling Diet Tips And Strategies That Work Fast!

I am extremely excited to pass this information along to you, and I am so happy that you now have read and can hopefully implement these strategies.

I hope this book was able to help you understand carb cycling and how to apply it to your daily routine to finally shed those pounds and build muscle.

The next step is to get started using this information and to hopefully live a healthy life!

Please don't be someone who just reads this information and doesn't apply it, the strategies in this book will only benefit you if you use them!

If you know of anyone else that could benefit from the information presented here please inform them of this book.

Finally, if you enjoyed this book and feel it has added value to your life in any way, please take the time to share your thoughts and post a review on Amazon. It'd be greatly appreciated!

Thank you and good luck!

Preview Of:

Low Carb Diet

The Best Guide To Low Carb - Lose Fat And Get A Fast Metabolism In 7 Days With This Weight Loss Blood Sugar Solution Diet!

Introduction

I want to thank you and congratulate you for purchasing the book, "Low Carb Diet: The Best Guide To Low Carb - Lose Fat And Get A Fast Metabolism In 7 Days With This Weight Loss Blood Sugar Solution Diet!".

This book contains proven steps and strategies on how to get the body of your dreams!

Don't let another week pass you by living life out of shape! The extra weight around your waistline or hips is more than just a problem of how you look in the mirror. Especially if it is not burned off in the near future, it can cause a host of other problems relating to your health and longevity. You owe it to yourself and the ones close to you to get in the best shape of your life.

Imagine how nice it would feel to look in the mirror and be happy with what you see on the outside and be comforted knowing that you are much healthier on the inside.

If you are serious about finally losing weight and keeping it off, then you have come to the right place. "Low Carb Diet: Low Carb Diet Solution - In as Little as 7 Days You Can Lose Weight Fast Using This Low Carb Diet Plan!" is the solution you have been looking for that allows you to literally create the body of your dreams, and what's even better is you will start seeing results within the first 7 days. Anyone who truly wants to lose weight can use these principles and be on their way in a matter of days! Don't waste another week, begin living life to the fullest today!

This book does not offer a drastic solution. But it will show you how to customize your low carb meals for seven days so you can start experiencing your desired weight loss results.

Thanks again for purchasing this book, I hope you enjoy it!

Chapter 1 – What Is A Low Carb Diet?

I am so excited for you! If you are reading this far, it means that you truly are looking for change in your life! You are tired of not living to your full potential, and ready to start living the way you were intended to. That's great, and what better way to start than by creating the best body of your life!

Keep that enthusiasm high because that is exactly what will carry you through to reaching your goals. The truth is the most important factor in your goals being obtained is you. You are the one that must "decide". You must simply make a choice that no matter what, you will reach your goal. If you simply do this, than I am confident you will succeed.

So let's get started! But Before we jump straight into what you should eat and the details of the diet, we need to make sure you are caught up to speed on the basics of a low carb diet.

If you've been dieting or have at least tried to do something about your weight, then you might have heard or read about low carb diets. Some of the popular fad-diets that can be classified as low carb diets include Sugar Busters Diet, the well-known South Beach Diet, the ever popular Zone Diet, Atkins, and pretty much every other diet you may have heard of.

As you should know by now, the term "low carb diet" has actually been applied to many different diets. It's a really broad classification of different diets that limit carbohydrate intake. Some people call them low glycemic diets while others refer to them as reduced carbohydrate diets.

The common denominator for these diets that belong to the "low carb" class is that they require, just as the name suggests, a diet that excludes foods that are heavy in carbohydrates. These are foods that are referred to as glycemic. There are lists of foods and their glycemic index to guide people going on any low carb diet.

So How Low Carb is Low Carb, Really?

You may consult your doctor about how low carb your diet should be; this is the smartest thing you should do before engaging in any diet. The dietary guidelines in the United States state that around 50 to 65 percent of a person's calorie intake for any given day should come from carbs.

Generally speaking, you should simply have less than 50% to 65% calories coming from carbohydrate sources of any variant in your daily diet. There are low carb diets that recommend only 20% or less of your daily caloric intake. If you want to live off a low carb diet for weight loss, keeping your carbohydrate intake to less than 20% of your daily caloric requirement is advised. Of course, you should make sure that you substitute this with another calorie source, mostly vegetables. With this kind of drastic drop in carbohydrate consumption, not all people are able to handle the dietary changes.

Your body will react. You can feel uneasy because of cravings for the carbs that you are used to having. That is why you will have to slowly adjust your carb intake up to the point when your body can take the loss of carbs. You may think that's a bit of a hit and miss approach, but the fact remains that everyone has a different tolerance for carb loss.

Thanks for Previewing My Exciting Book Entitled:

"Low Carb Diet: The Best Guide To Low Carb - Lose Fat And Get A Fast Metabolism In 7 Days With This Weight Loss Blood Sugar Solution Diet!"

To purchase this book, simply go to the Amazon Kindle store and simply search:

"LOW CARB DIET"

Then just scroll down until you see my book. You will know it is mine because you will see my name "Chris Smith" underneath the title.

Alternatively, you can visit my author page on Amazon to see this book and other work I have done. Thanks so much, and please don't forget your free bonuses

DON'T LEAVE YET! - CHECK OUT YOUR FREE BONUSES BELOW!

Free Bonus Offer: Get Free Access To The LiveFitVIP.com VIP Newsletter!

Once you enter your email address you will immediately get free access to this awesome newsletter!

But wait, right now if you join now for free you will also get free access to the "The 7 Keys To Body Transformation" free EBook!

To claim both your FREE VIP NEWSLETTER MEMBERSHIP and your FREE BONUS EBook on THE 7 KEYS TO BODY TRANSFORMATION!

Just Go To:

www.liveFitVIP.com

www.ingramcontent.com/pod-product-compliance
Lightning Source LLC
Chambersburg PA
CBHW070935290526
45795CB00003B/1025